Let's Listen, Speak and Learn

# 臨床看護英語

第6版

仁木 久恵　聖路加国際大学　名誉教授
Nancy Sharts-Hopko　ヴィラノヴァ大学看護学部　教授
横田 まり子　東京医科大学　兼任講師

医学書院

Let's Listen, Speak and Learn
臨床看護英語

| 発　行 | 1986 年 4 月 1 日 | 第 1 版第 1 刷 |
|---|---|---|
| | 1989 年 5 月 1 日 | 第 1 版第 5 刷 |
| | 1990 年 4 月 1 日 | 新訂版第 1 刷 |
| | 1996 年 3 月15日 | 新訂版第10刷 |
| | 1997 年 7 月 1 日 | 第 3 版第 1 刷 |
| | 2000 年12月 1 日 | 第 3 版第 5 刷 |
| | 2001 年10月15日 | 第 4 版第 1 刷 |
| | 2011 年 2 月 1 日 | 第 4 版第10刷 |
| | 2012 年 7 月15日 | 第 5 版第 1 刷 |
| | 2018 年10月15日 | 第 5 版第 5 刷 |
| | 2020 年10月15日 | 第 6 版第 1 刷Ⓒ |
| | 2022 年12月 1 日 | 第 6 版第 2 刷 |

著　者　仁木久恵 ナンシー・シャーツ-ホプコ
　　　　横田まり子

発行者　株式会社　医学書院
　　　　代表取締役　金原　俊
　　　　〒113-8719　東京都文京区本郷 1-28-23
　　　　電話　03-3817-5600(社内案内)

組　版　ビーコム
印刷・製本　三報社印刷

本書の複製権・翻訳権・上映権・譲渡権・貸与権・公衆送信権(送信可能化権を含む)は株式会社医学書院が保有します.

ISBN978-4-260-04198-0

# はじめに

　日本を訪れる外国人は近年増加しており，また日本で暮らす外国人の数も増え続けるでしょう．病気になれば誰しも不安にかられますが，日本に滞在中の外国人が体調を崩したり，けがをしたとき，彼らと直に接する看護師の役割は重大です．英語をマスターすることで，患者さんから多くの情報を得るばかりでなく，よりよい信頼関係を築くことができます．今後，英語を話せる看護師は貴重な存在として，その活躍の場が増え続けることでしょう．

　本書はそんなニーズに応えて編まれたテキストです．臨床の現場で起こり得るさまざまな状況を想定して，「すぐに使える英語表現」が着実に身につくように工夫しています．

　改訂するにあたって，最新の情報や知見を取り入れて大幅に加筆・修正しました．本書の最大の特徴は「学習者中心」の視点に立っており，耳で聴く（Let's Listen），発音練習をする（Pronunciation），主体的に話す（Let's Speak），そして看護に関連する表現や語彙を増やす（Let's Learn）で構成されています．とりわけ今回は，会話（Let's Speak）に重点を置いて改訂しました．また，Nursing Tip のコラムを設けて，知っておくと役立つ情報も幅広く取り上げています．新たに，語彙の索引を巻末につけました．本書で紹介している患者さんの視点にたった会話表現を練習することによって，いざというときにもスムーズに対応することができるような英語力をつけてください．

　なお，英語音声データを医学書院の Web ページに用意しました．本書をより効果的に活用できるように Let's Listen, Pronunciation, Let's Learn を収録しましたので，下記の URL にアクセスして，ID（igakurinsho），パスワード（kangoeigo6）を入力のうえ英語音声の無料ダウンロードをご利用ください（http://www.igaku-shoin.co.jp/prd/04198/audio/）．

　最後に，初版からご尽力くださった聖路加国際大学名誉教授の助川尚子氏に心からの謝意を表します．

著者を代表して　仁木久恵

# 各 Chapter の構成と効果的な学習法

　本書の題材は，看護を専門とする方々が臨床の場で出会うコミュニケーション状況を想定して選んだものです．「Let's Listen」「Let's Speak」「Let's Learn」の3部に分かれており，臨床看護の英語表現として最小限必要と思われる基本文型と語彙を提示しています．

## Let's Listen

**MODEL DIALOGUE**：自然な英文を何度も聴いて，状況にあった表現をインプットします．英語的な発想に慣れてください．語句の注は最小限にとどめてありますので，必要に応じて巻末の語彙索引を参照してください．

**PRONUNCIATION**：モデルの発音，イントネーションをよく聴いて，あとについて必ず声に出して練習してください．音の強弱によって英語特有のリズムが生まれます．また，音と音の重なり，脱落などにも注意してください．皆さんは，自分の声を自分の耳で聴くことによって，いっそう「聴く力」がつき，次のステップ「話す」ことにも自信がもてるようになるはずです．テキストを閉じモデルの声について，正しい発音で言えるようになるまで練習を繰り返してください．

**NOTES**：臨床看護の英文によく出てくる基本文型や語彙を中心に説明してあります．

## Let's Speak

　これまで学んだ表現や語彙を実際に使って，ペアを組んで会話をします．文法上の細かな誤りはあまり気にせず，リラックスした雰囲気で会話してください．ペアの相手は，1か月に一度は替えるなどの工夫をしましょう．

## Let's Learn

　身体部位の英語名など看護に関連する語彙や慣用句を学びます．また，接頭辞・接尾辞を覚えながら造語システムを学ぶことによって，語彙が豊富になり，英語の理解力が飛躍的に伸びるでしょう．

# 目次

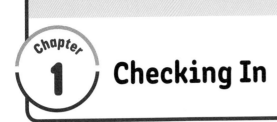

# Checking In

## Let's Listen

*Mr. McKay visits Tokyo International Hospital for the first time. Ms. Hosoda is a nurse.*

**Nurse**  Good morning. I'm Nurse Hosoda. May I help you?

**Patient**  Hello. I have a terrible headache.

**Nurse**  Is this your first visit?

**Patient**  Yes, it is.

**Nurse**  Do you have a referral letter?

**Patient**  No, I don't.

**Nurse**  Then, please fill out this form. Write in block letters*, please.

**Patient**  OK.

......

**Patient**  I'm finished. Here it is.

**Nurse**  Do you have Japanese health insurance?

**Patient**  Yes. Here's my card.

**Nurse**  How do you pronounce your last name?

**Patient**  McKay.

**Nurse**  I beg your pardon?

**Patient**  MC・KAY.

**Nurse**  Thank you, Mr. McKay. Please wait here until we call your name.

**Patient**  Sure.

---

\* in block letters：大文字の活字体で.

1. núrse    2. pátient    3. térrible héadache    4. fírst vísit

5. reférral lètter    6. fíll óut    7. phóne nùmber    8. áddress

9. occupátion    10. May I help you?

11. Do you have Japanese health insurance?    12. I beg your pardon?

13. How do you pronounce your last name?

14. Please wait here until we call your name.

15. Tell me the date of your birth.

## NOTES

1. 発音の確認・聞き返すときの表現

    (1) 名前をどのように発音するかを確認するとき

    How do you pronounce your last name*?
    姓(名字)はどのように発音するのですか.

    (2) 聞き取れなかったとき　❶最後を上げる

    I beg your pardon?／Pardon me?／Could you please say it again?
    もう一度言ってください.

    Could you speak more slowly, please?
    もっとゆっくり話してください.

2. 住所の読み方・書き方

    日本とは逆に小さい番地から大きな地名へと読む.

    423 Third Street, Larchmont, California 97189

    ❶数字は four twenty-three [four two three] と読む. 97189 は郵便番号 (postal code/zip code) で, nine-seven-one-eight-nine と読む.

    4-42-12 Kita-Ogikubo, Suginami-ku, Tokyo 167-0052

    ❶数字は four, forty-two, twelve と読む. 4丁目42番地12号は, 42-12, 4-chome でもよい.

---

* family name とも言う.

### 3. 電話番号の読み方

My mobile phone number is 090-3392-4867.

❹ 0*-nine-zero, three-three-nine-two, four-eight-six-seven と読む.

### 4. WH 疑問文

What, Who, When, Where, How などで始まる疑問文は，ふつう文の最後を下げるが，親しみの気持ちを表すときには上げ調子で言うこともある.

❹ What's your name?↗  この文を下げ調子で言うと「名前を言いなさい」と威圧するような強い口調になる.

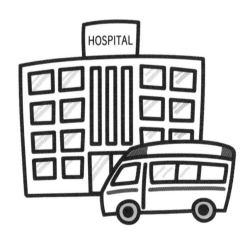

---

\* 0[zíːrou／ou]

**A.** *Work in pairs and practice the dialogue on page 1. When you become the nurse, please try to close the textbook.*

. . . . . . . . . . . . . . . . . . . . . . . . . . . . . . . . . . . . . . . . . . . . . . . . . . . . . . . . . . . . . . . . . . . . . . .

**B.** *Interview your partner and obtain some information to fill out the following chart. While you are asking questions, your partner should close her/his textbook. After you have finished, exchange roles with her/him.*

1. Partner's Name : _____

2. Phone number : (Home)_____ (Mobile)_____

3. Address :

   _____

   (e.g. 3-2-5 Yamate, Naka-ku, Yokohama-shi, Kanagawa 225-0001)

4. Date of Birth : _____ (e.g. Sept. 7, 2001)

5. Place of Birth : _____ (e.g. Kobe, Hyogo)

6. Occupation : ☐ business person  ☐ self-employed  ☐ student  ☐ other :

   _____

   (e.g. She/He works for an IT company./She/He is a nursing student.)

7. Referral Letter : ☐ Yes  ☐ No

8. Japanese Health Insurance : ☐ Yes  ☐ No

9. Chief Complaint : _____

   ☐ a headache  ☐ a high fever  ☐ trouble breathing  ☐ _____

   (e.g. She/He has a headache./She/He has trouble breathing. )

10. Any Other Information : _____

    (e.g. She/He lives with her/his roommate./She/He returned from India yesterday.)

Tokyo International Hospital

## Registration Form

Date：2021/9/15

Name：*WARD Mary** ☐ Mr. ☐ Ms. ☑ Mrs. ☐ Miss

Gender：☐ male ☑ female ☐ non-binary ☐ prefer not to answer

Date of Birth：*1987/9/4* Age：*34* years old

Current Address：
*Sunny Place #312, 1-3-5 Aoyama, Minato-ku, Tokyo 108-0071*

Phone Home：*03-3411-xxxx*
Mobile：*090-9140-xxxx*

Nationality：*American* Native Language：*English*

Occupation：*teacher of English* Religion：*Catholic*

Do you have Japanese health insurance?
☑ Yes ☐ No

Do you have a referral letter?
☐ Yes ☑ No

Do you have an appointment?
☐ Yes ☑ No

Emergency Contact Number：
Home：*the same as above* Mobile：*090-5123-xxxx*
Name：*WARD Peter* Relationship：*husband*

Any Other Information：
*stomachache / nausea / request for an interpreter*

---

\* 日本の病院なので，名前や生年月日は日本式に姓，名の順で書く．姓は大文字で．

*Imagine that you are John Lewis from Toronto. Fill out the chart on the next page, based on the data below.*

氏名：John Lewis
生年月日：1958 年 12 月 18 日　　○歳
現住所：東京都文京区本郷 1-28-23　　郵便番号：113-0033
固定電話：03-3817-××××　　　　携帯電話：090-7834-××××
国籍：カナダ(Canadian)　　　　　母語：英語
職業：銀行員(bank clerk)　　　　　宗教：プロテスタント(Protestant)
保険：国民健康保険
紹介状：なし
予約：なし
緊急連絡先：固定電話：03-3817-××××
　　　　　　携帯電話：090-2358-××××
　　　　　　氏名・続柄：Karen Lewis, wife
主訴：高熱(high fever)，咳(cough)，胸痛(chest pain)

# Registration Form

Date ： _____
year / month / day

| | |
|---|---|
| Name ： _____ ☐ Mr.   ☐ Ms.   ☐ Mrs.   ☐ Miss<br>     last / first / middle | |
| Gender ： ☐ male    ☐ female    ☐ non-binary    ☐ prefer not to answer | |
| Date of Birth ： _____<br>    year / month / day | Age ： _____ years old |
| Current Address ： _____<br>_____<br>house number / street / ward / city / postal code | Phone Home ：<br>Mobile ： |
| Nationality ： | Native Language ： |
| Occupation ： | Religion ： |
| Do you have Japanese health insurance?<br>☐ Yes    ☐ No | |
| Do you have a referral letter?<br>☐ Yes    ☐ No | |
| Do you have an appointment?<br>☐ Yes    ☐ No | |
| Emergency Contact Number ：<br>  Home ：               Mobile ：<br>  Name ：              Relationship ： | |
| Any Other Information ： | |

1. Nationality（国籍）を尋ねるとき　What's your nationality?

Américan　アメリカ人，米国人　　Canádian　カナダ人

Chinése　中国人　　　　　　　　Frénch　フランス人

Gérman　ドイツ人　　　　　　　Índian　インド人

Koréan　韓国人，朝鮮人　　　　　Rússian　ロシア人

❶ イギリス（the United Kingdom［U.K.］）の場合は一括して Brítish（イギリス人，英国人）と言うが，その人の出身地によって次のようにも言う. Énglish　イングランド人，Scóttish　スコットランド人，Írish　アイルランド人，Wélsh　ウェールズ人.

2. Religion（宗教）を尋ねるとき　What's your religion?

❶ 質問が唐突にならないよう，前もって Are you religious? などと尋ねるとよい.

Christiánity　キリスト教　　　　　Chrístian　キリスト教徒

　Cathólicism　カトリック教　　　　Cátholic　カトリック教徒

　Prótestantism　プロテスタント（新教）　Prótestant　プロテスタント教徒

Júdaism　ユダヤ教　　　　　　　Jéwish pèrson　ユダヤ教徒

　　　　　　　　　　　　　　　　❶ Jew は差別的な響きがあるので避けたい.

Íslam　イスラム教　　　　　　　Múslim　イスラム教徒

Jehòvah's Wítnesses　エホバの証人

Jehòvah's Wítness　エホバの証人の信徒

❶ 世界に宗教団体は数限りなくあるため，ほかの宗教という意味で other と書いてもよい. あるいは，特定の宗教をもたない場合には none と書く.

3. Marital status（婚姻状態）を尋ねるとき　What's your marital status?

síngle　独身（の）

márried　結婚している

wídowed　妻［夫］を亡くしている

divórced　離婚している

séparated　別居している

líving with pártner　パートナーと暮らしている

# General Consultation

## 🔊 Let's Listen

*Kate Anson, a university student, needs to see a doctor for abdominal pain.*
*Nurse Sato is obtaining information about her problem.*

| | |
|---|---|
| **Nurse** | Hello, Ms. Anson. I'm Nurse Sato. Please have a seat. How can I help you today? |
| **Ms. Anson** | I have some pain in my abdomen. |
| **Nurse** | How long have you had the pain? |
| **Ms. Anson** | About two days. |
| **Nurse** | What kind of pain is it? |
| **Ms. Anson** | It's really sharp. It hurts very badly. |
| **Nurse** | Where is the pain? |
| **Ms. Anson** | Well, … around here, in my lower abdomen. |
| **Nurse** | Do you have any other symptoms? |
| **Ms. Anson** | I also have nausea. I vomited this morning. |
| **Nurse** | Do you have a fever? |
| **Ms. Anson** | Yes, I have a slight fever. |
| **Nurse** | Now, go to the department of surgery. One of our staff will take you there. |
| **Ms. Anson** | Thank you. |

1. ábdomen    2. náusea    3. súrgery    4. hígh féver    5. thróat

6. báck    7. áche    8. dúll pàin    9. thróbbing páin    10. vómit

11. How can I help you?    12. I have some pain in my abdomen.

13. What kind of pain is it?    14. Where is the pain?

15. Do you have any other symptoms?

16. How long have you had the problem?

17. How did it start?    18. Go to the department of Internal Medicine.

## NOTES

1. 痛みの表現

　　pain は一般的な痛みを表し，ache は通例，身体の一部に継続的に感じる鈍痛を表す．身体各部の痛みについては，痛む部位のあとに続けて合成語を形成することが多い．〔例〕headache, stomachache, toothache. また「痛む」という場合は，have pain（an ache），feel pain（an ache）として用いる．

　　痛みの程度を表すには, a mild pain（軽い痛み），a severe pain（ひどい痛み）のように修飾語をつける．hurt は主として外部から心身に与えられた痛みで，動詞として使うことが多い．

2. 症状について患者に尋ねる

　（1）What kind of problem is it?　どんな症状ですか．（症状の特徴）

　　　How severe is it?　程度はどのくらいですか．（症状の程度）

　（2）Where is it?　場所はどこですか．（症状の部位）

　　　Please show me where you have the pain.

　　　どこが痛むのか教えてください．

　（3）When did it start?　いつからですか．（発症時刻・時期）

　　　How did it occur?　どのように起こりましたか．（症状の起こり方）

　　　Did it come on suddenly or slowly?　突然でしたか，徐々にでしたか．

　（4）How long have you had the problem?

　　　どのくらい続いていますか．（症状の継続時間）

(5) Do you have any other symptoms?

　　ほかに何か症状がありますか.（随伴症状）

## 3. 痛みの程度を尋ねる

Please look at the scale of zero to ten. What's your pain level now?

痛みの強さ(0～10)を表すスケールをご覧ください.　今の痛みのレベルはど

のあたりですか.

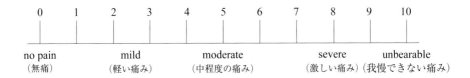

*Choose either "influenza" or "appendicitis" (you and your partner should not choose the same disease). Then, ask her/him about her/his problem. Fill out the chart below. After you have finished, exchange roles with her/him.*

Conversation starter：A：How can I help you today?　B：I have a terrible pain.

1.  Site*：She/He has a (terrible) pain in her/his (　　　　　　　　).

     ☐ throat　☐ back　☐ chest　☐ abdomen　☐ _____

2.  Character of the pain：It's a (　　　　　　　　) pain.

     ☐ dull　☐ sharp　☐ shooting　☐ throbbing　☐ _____

3.  Onset**：It started (　　　　　　　　).

     ☐ suddenly　☐ slowly

4.  Duration：She/He has had the pain (　　　　　　　　).

     ☐ since last night　☐ for three days　☐ for a week　☐ _____

5.  Other symptoms：She/He has (　　　　　　　　).

     ☐ nausea　☐ loose bowel movements　☐ vomiting　☐ a high fever

     ☐ _____

6.  Any other information：_____

     (Speak freely.) (e.g. She/He couldn't sleep all night.／Her/His whole body aches.)

7.  Clinical department：She/He should go to the department of _____.

     ☐ Surgery　☐ Internal Medicine　☐ _____

---

\* 体の部位.　　\*\* 病気などの始まり.

## Clinical Department

Géneral Médicine*　総合診療科

Intérnal Médicine　内科

　Réspiratory Médicine　呼吸器内科

　Cardiólogy　循環器内科

　Gastroenterólogy　消化器内科

　Metábolism and Endocrinólogy　代謝・内分泌内科

　Nephrólogy　腎臓内科

　Neurólogy［Néuroscience］　神経内科

　Hematólogy　血液内科

　Rheumatólogy/Immunólogy and Állergy　リウマチ/免疫・アレルギー内科

　Geriátrics　老年内科

　Psychosomátic Médicine　心療内科

　Oncólogy　腫瘍内科

Súrgery　外科

　Géneral Súrgery　一般外科

　Cardiováscular Súrgery　心臓血管外科

　Thorácic Súrgery　呼吸器外科

　Gastroenterológical Súrgery　消化器外科

　Bréast and Éndocrine Súrgery　乳腺・内分泌外科

　Néurosurgery　脳神経外科

　Orthopédic Súrgery［Orthopédics］　整形外科

　Pediátric Súrgery　小児外科

　Plástic Súrgery　形成外科

Pediátrics　小児科

Obstétrics　産科

Gynecólogy　婦人科

---

\* 紹介状を持たずに来院し，どの科を受診すればよいかわからない初診患者が最初にかかると
ころ．

13

Urólogy　泌尿器科

Psychíatry　精神科

Ophthalmólogy　眼科

Ótorhinolaryngólogy〔ENT（Ear, Nose, and Throat）〕　耳鼻咽喉科

Dermatólogy　皮膚科

Pálliative Cáre　緩和ケア科

Radiólogy　放射線科

Anesthesiólogy　麻酔科

Diagnóstic Pathólogy　病理診断科

Déntistry　歯科

　　Óral（and Maxillofácial）Súrgery　口腔外科

Médical Genétics　遺伝子診断科

Emérgency and Crítical Cáre　救急部

Rehabilitátion　リハビリテーション科

Comprehénsive Phýsical Examinàtion〔Héalth Scréening〕Cènter
　　人間ドック・健診センター

*Which department would you visit…*

1. when a child is sick?      P _____

2. when someone breaks an ankle?      O _____

3. when you get a rash?      D _____

4. when you have a pain in your eyes?      O _____

5. when someone is having a baby?      O _____

6. when a friend has a severe toothache?      D _____

7. when someone gets seriously injured in a motorcycle accident?

     E _____

8. when your grandfather has shortness of breath and a pain in the chest?

     C _____

9. when someone needs to be put to sleep for surgery?      A _____

10. when the lump in your breast feels firm, and it has an irregular shape and size?

     B _____

nurse*　看護師

associate nurse, assistant nurse　准看護師

nursing assistant, nurse's aide　看護助手

nursing student　看護学生

director of nursing　看護部長

nursing supervisor　看護師長

charge nurse, head nurse　主任看護師，看護主任

outpatient nurse　外来看護師

floor nurse, staff nurse　病棟看護師

surgical nurse, scrub nurse　手術室看護師

midwife　助産師

visiting nurse　訪問看護師

public health nurse［PHN］　保健師

school nurse　養護教諭，（大学などの）学校保健師

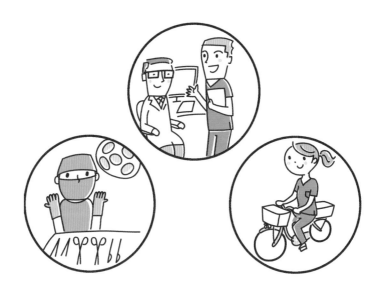

---

\* 上級看護師としては nurse practitioner（ナース・プラクティショナー），certified nurse（認定看護師），（clinical）nurse specialist（専門看護師）がある．

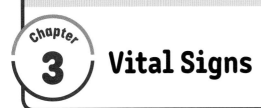

# Vital Signs

## Chapter 3

## Let's Listen

*Nurse Ichiro Kita is taking Mrs. Kim's vital signs.*

**Nurse**     Good morning, Mrs. Kim. My name is Ichiro Kita.

**Mrs. Kim**   Hello, Nurse.

**Nurse**     Let me take your temperature. Please keep this thermometer under your arm until it beeps.

**Mrs. Kim**   OK.

**Nurse**     I'm going to place this pulse oximeter on your finger to measure your pulse and oxygen level.

       ......

**Nurse**     Your temperature is 37.1 degrees Celsius. Do you have a headache?

**Mrs. Kim**   Well, yes, a little, but not so bad.

**Nurse**     Did you sleep well last night?

**Mrs. Kim**   Yes, I did. I slept like a baby.

**Nurse**     Fine. Now I'd like to check your blood pressure. Hold out your left arm and roll up your sleeve, please … now, relax your arm.

       ......

**Nurse**     Your blood pressure is 128 over 84*.

**Mrs. Kim**   That's very good, for me.

---

\* 収縮期血圧 128, 拡張期血圧 84 を表す.

1. vítal sígns    2. témperature    3. thermómeter    4. púlse oxímeter

5. óxygen lèvel    6. méasure    7. 37.1 degrées Célsius

8. blóod prèssure    9. reláx

10. Let me take your temperature.

11. Please keep this thermometer under your arm until it beeps.

12. I'm going to place this pulse oximeter on your finger.

13. I'd like to check your blood pressure.

## NOTES

1. take *one's* vital signs　バイタルサインを調べる

   ❶ take（check, measure）を用いて「〜を測る（調べる）」の意味を表すことがで
   きる．take *one's* blood pressure　血圧を測る / take *one's* pulse　脈拍を測
   る / take *one's* temperature　検温する，など．

2. 自分がこれから行おうとしていることについて相手にその意向を伝える場合

   （1）*I'm going* to make you a little more comfortable.
   　　もう少し楽にしてあげましょう．

   （2）*I'll* check with Dr. Hayashi.　林先生に伺って確かめてみましょう．

   （3）*Let me* fluff your pillow.　枕をふくらませましょう．

   （4）*I'd like* to ask you some questions.
   　　少しお伺いしたいことがあるのですが．

   ❶ (1)(2)(3)は同じように「〜しましょう」という意思表現であるが，(3)は婉
   曲的でやわらかい．(4)は「できれば」というニュアンスを含んだ，さらに婉
   曲的で丁寧な意思の表現．

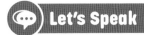

## Let's Speak

*You are going to take your partner's vital signs. Please follow the three steps below. Use the following expressions for a nurse, while your partner is using the ones for a patient. After you have finished, exchange roles with her/him.*

[a nurse] I'd like to _____./First let me _____./

Next I'm going to _____./Then I'll _____./

Please keep this thermometer under..../Hold out your left arm and....

Your temperature/blood pressure is....

(That's normal./A little high, but don't worry.)

[a patient] OK./Yes./That's good for me./A little high/low./Is that normal?

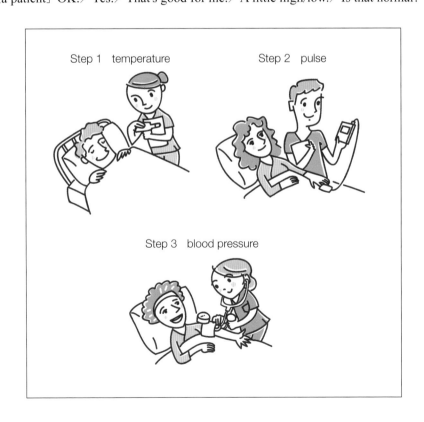

Step 1   temperature

Step 2   pulse

Step 3   blood pressure

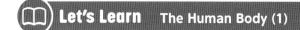

**Let's Learn** The Human Body (1)

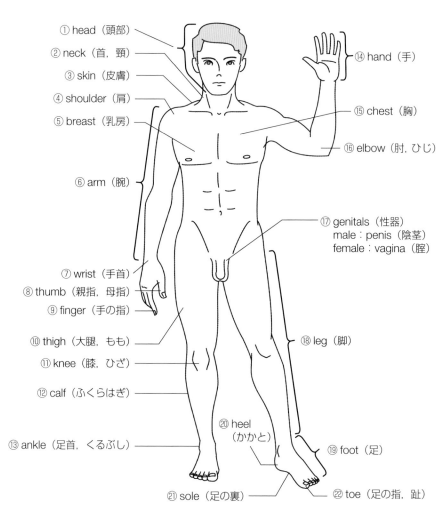

EXTERNAL（外部）

male（男性）　female（女性）

① head（頭部）

② neck（首，頸）

③ skin（皮膚）

④ shoulder（肩）

⑤ breast（乳房）

⑥ arm（腕）

⑦ wrist（手首）

⑧ thumb（親指，母指）

⑨ finger（手の指）

⑩ thigh（大腿，もも）

⑪ knee（膝，ひざ）

⑫ calf（ふくらはぎ）

⑬ ankle（足首，くるぶし）

⑭ hand（手）

⑮ chest（胸）

⑯ elbow（肘，ひじ）

⑰ genitals（性器）
male：penis（陰茎）
female：vagina（腟）

⑱ leg（脚）

⑲ foot（足）

⑳ heel（かかと）

㉑ sole（足の裏）

㉒ toe（足の指，趾）

## EXERCISE

*Fill in the blanks.*

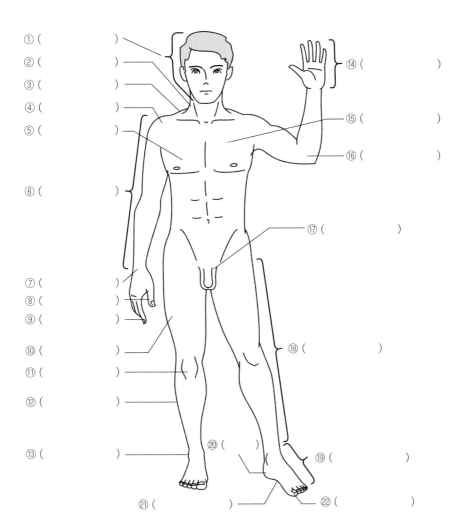

① (        )

② (        )

③ (        )

④ (        )

⑤ (        )

⑥ (        )

⑦ (        )

⑧ (        )

⑨ (        )

⑩ (        )

⑪ (        )

⑫ (        )

⑬ (        )

⑭ (        )

⑮ (        )

⑯ (        )

⑰ (        )

⑱ (        )

⑲ (        )

⑳ (        )

㉑ (        )

㉒ (        )

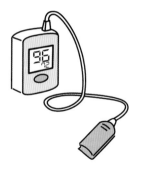

pulse oximeter (パルスオキシメーター)

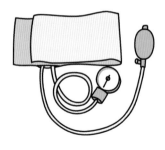

blood pressure monitor (血圧計)
❗ sphygmomanometer とも言う.

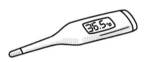

thermometer (体温計)

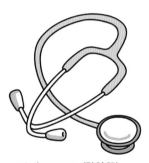

stethoscope (聴診器)

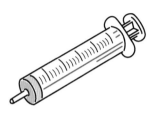

syringe (注射器)

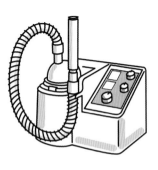

nebulizer (ネブライザー)

# Admission and Orientation to the Hospital Routine

 **Let's Listen**

*Nurse Wada is showing Mrs. Cohen around her room at Tokyo International Hospital.*

| | |
|---|---|
| **Nurse** | Hi, Mrs. Cohen. I'm Nurse Wada. Let me show you around the room. |
| **Mrs. Cohen** | Oh, thank you. |
| **Nurse** | This is your bed, and this is your bedside table. The nurse call bell is here by the pillow. |
| **Mrs. Cohen** | How does it work? |
| **Nurse** | Just push this button, and the nurse will come to see what you need. |
| **Mrs. Cohen** | Where can I put my things? |
| **Nurse** | Here's your locker, and that one is for your roommate. You can also use the bedside table. |
| **Mrs. Cohen** | What's the schedule of meals? |
| **Nurse** | Breakfast is served at 8:00 o'clock, lunch is at noon, and dinner is at 6:00 o'clock. And lights-out is at 9:00 o'clock. If you have any questions, let us know. |
| **Mrs. Cohen** | OK. Thank you. |
| **Nurse** | You're welcome. |

1. bédside tàble     2. núrse cáll bèll     3. lócker     4. hóspital gòwn

5. óverbed tàble     6. IV́ stànd     7. óxygen óutlet

8. This is your bed.     9. That one is for your roommate.

10. The nurse call bell is here by the pillow.

11. Just push this button, and the nurse will come to see what you need.

12. If you have any questions, please let us know.

Patient Room(病室)

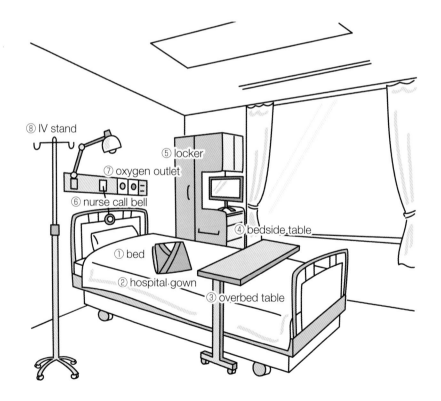

⑧ IV stand

⑤ locker

⑦ oxygen outlet

⑥ nurse call bell

④ bedside table

① bed

② hospital gown

③ overbed table

## 🗣 Let's Speak

*Show your partner around the patient room, pointing to items in the picture. Use the following expressions for a nurse and the questions for a patient. Take turns.*

⟨You⟩

This is ..../Here's ..../That is ....

It's right here/there ....

You can use/wear ....

Please push/put/use ....

⟨Your partner⟩

What is this/that?

Where is...?

Where can I put...?

How does it work?

Conversation starter：

A：Hi,_____ I'm Nurse _____.
        ⟨partner's name⟩                    ⟨your name⟩

    Let me show you around the room. This is _____.

B：OK. What is this?

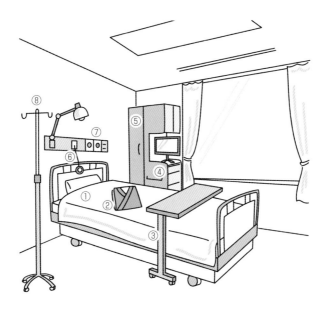

## Hospital Unit

médical flòor　内科病棟
　❶ ward［unit］とも言う.
súrgical flòor　外科病棟
pediátric flòor　小児科病棟
orthopédic flòor　整形外科病棟
gynecológical flòor　婦人科病棟
matérnity flòor　産科病棟
　lábor ròom　陣痛室
　delívery ròom　分娩室
　recóvery ròom　回復室
　núrsery　新生児室
pálliative cáre ùnit［PCU］
　緩和ケア病棟
inténsive cáre ùnit［ICU］
　集中治療室(部),集中ケア病棟
córonary cáre ùnit［CCU］
　冠疾患集中治療室(部)
núrses' stàtion　ナースステーション
ínterview ròom　面談室
pátient ròom　病室
　prívate ròom　個室
　sèmi-prívate ròom　2人部屋
　fóur-bèd ròom　4人部屋
pátients' lóunge　患者用ラウンジ
wáiting ròom　待合室
intérnal médicine óutpatient
　depàrtment　内科外来
súrgery óutpatient depàrtment
　外科外来

consultátion ròom［dóctor's òffice］
　診察室
　❶ examination room とも言う.
emérgency ròom［ER］
　救急外来,救急室
láboratory　検査室
óperating ròom［OR］　手術室
phármacy　薬局
cafetéria　カフェテリア,食堂
hóspital［gíft］shòp　売店

1st flòor　1階
2nd flòor　2階
3rd flòor　3階
4th flòor　4階
5th flòor　5階
básement　地下

26

*Where's Ms. Yamada working?*

She's taking care of ...

1. a sick child                                               on a _____ floor.

2. a mother who has just given birth to a boy    on a _____ floor.

3. a man who has had an automobile accident    in an _____ room.

4. a girl who had a broken leg                        on an _____ floor.

5. a woman with pneumonia                           on a _____ floor.

6. a man who had an appendectomy yesterday    on a _____ floor.

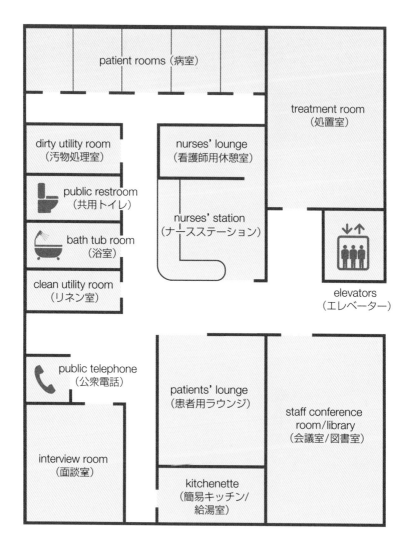

## Chapter 5

# Data Collection from Patients

*Nurse Suzuki is obtaining information about his problem from Ted Jones, a middle-aged businessman.*

**Nurse** I see you're here because you have chest pain, is that right?

**Mr. Jones** Yes, I also have trouble breathing.

**Nurse** How long have you had these problems?

**Mr. Jones** About two weeks.

**Nurse** Have you taken any medications?

**Mr. Jones** Yes, I took painkillers, but they didn't help.

**Nurse** Are you having any difficulty sleeping?

**Mr. Jones** Yes. I couldn't sleep last night.

**Nurse** How's your appetite?

**Mr. Jones** Not very good. I don't feel like eating.

**Nurse** Are you having regular bowel movements?

**Mr. Jones** Yes. No problem there.

**Nurse** Do you smoke?

**Mr. Jones** No, I quit three years ago, and haven't smoked since then.

**Nurse** Do you have any allergies?

**Mr. Jones** No, I don't.

1. próblem    2. tróuble bréathing    3. páinkiller    4. állergies    5. póllen

6. cóugh    7. rásh on the fáce    8. dízziness

9. lóose bówel mòvements    10. cónstipated    11. antibiótics    12. láxative

13. Have you táken any medicátions?    14. Hów's your appetite?

15. Are you háving régular bówel movements?

16. Do you háve any állergies?    17. She is allérgic to dúst.

1. How can I help you?

「どうしましたか」に相当する表現で，診療所や病院を訪れた人に対して医師や看護師がする質問. What's the matter with you?／What can I do for you? も同様に用いられる.

2. Have you noticed any other changes?

ほかに何か気づいたことはありませんか.

「have + 過去分詞」は現在完了形を形成し，以下のような意味を表す.

(1)「もう〜してしまった」(完了)

Have you taken your medications?　薬を飲みましたか.

(2)「今まで〜したことがある」(経験)

I've [have] been in the hospital before.　以前入院したことがある.

(3)「(過去のある時から)今までずっと〜している」(継続)

How long have you had this problem?

この状態はどのくらい続いていますか.

(4)「ある動作の結果〜である」(結果)

The patient has gone to the X-ray department.

患者はレントゲン室に行って今ここにいない.

# 🗨 Let's Speak

*First, read through the chart below and put checks in the boxes you choose.*
*Then, imagine that you (nurse) are asking questions to your partner (patient)*
*about her/his problems to get some necessary clinical data. While you are*
*asking, put checks in the partner's boxes. After you have finished, exchange*
*roles with her/him.*

Conversation starter : How can I help you today?／What's the matter with you?

You　　Your partner (Name _____)

1. Problem :

　□　　□　　A (slight/terrible) pain in the stomach.
　□　　□　　A (slight/terrible) headache.
　□　　□　　Nausea.
　□　　□　　A cough.
　□　　□　　Difficulty sleeping.

2. Other Symptoms :

　□　　□　　A back pain.
　□　　□　　A rash on the face.
　□　　□　　Dizziness.
　□　　□　　_____.

3. Duration :

　□　　□　　Since last night.
　□　　□　　For three days.
　□　　□　　For a week.
　□　　□　　For more than a week.
　□　　□　　_____.

4. Fever :

　□　　□　　Yes, _____ degrees Celsius.
　□　　□　　No, but I feel [she/he feels] feverish.
　□　　□　　No.

31

5. Appetite：
   ☐　　☐　　No appetite.
   ☐　　☐　　A little appetite.
   ☐　　☐　　OK.
6. Bowel Movements：
   ☐　　☐　　Yes, regular.
   ☐　　☐　　No, I have [she/he has] loose bowel movements.
   ☐　　☐　　No, I have [she/he has] been constipated.
7. Medications：
   ☐　　☐　　Yes, I [she/he] took _____ .
   　　　　　　(e.g. sleeping pills, painkillers, laxatives, antibiotics)
   ☐　　☐　　No.
8. Allergies：
   ☐　　☐　　Yes, I am [she/he is] allergic to _____ .
   　　　　　　(e.g. pollen, eggs, insects, cosmetics, antibiotics, dust)
   ☐　　☐　　No.
   (If yes,) how often do you have an allergic reaction?：
   ☐　　☐　　Only at certain times of the year.
   ☐　　☐　　All the time.
   What happens when you have [she/he has] an allergic reaction?
   ☐　　☐　　A rash.
   ☐　　☐　　Swelling.
   ☐　　☐　　Itchy eyes.
   ☐　　☐　　Difficulty breathing.
   ☐　　☐　　Anaphylactic shock.
Any Other Information：
   ☐　　☐　　_____
(Speak freely.)

**Let's Learn**

Severity and Types of Pain

◆ 痛みの程度を示す表現　How severe is the pain?

nó pàin　痛みなし

míld [slíght] pàin　軽い[少しの]痛み

tólerable pàin　我慢できる程度の痛み

móderate pàin　中程度の痛み

sevére pàin　激しい[強い]痛み

unbéarable pàin　耐えられない痛み

◆ 痛みの性質や種類を表す一般的な表現

áche　継続的な鈍い痛み，うずき（動詞：うずく）

acúte pàin　急性の痛み

búrning pàin　焼けつくような痛み，灼熱痛

chrónic pàin　慢性の痛み，慢性疼痛

cónstant pàin　持続的な痛み

crámpy pàin　けいれん性のひきつるような痛み

déep pàin　深部の痛み

dúll pàin　鈍痛，鈍い痛み

géneralized pàin　全身[広範性]の痛み

grádual pàin　徐々に出る痛み

lócalized pàin　局所[限局性]の痛み

periódic pàin　周期性の痛み

príckly pàin, tíngling pàin　チクチクする痛み

rádiating pàin　放散性の痛み

shárp pàin　鋭い痛み

shóoting pàin　ビーンと走るような鋭い痛み

sóreness　（炎症・傷などの）ヒリヒリする痛み

stíffness　（体の部位の）凝った痛み

súdden pàin　突発性の痛み

superfícial pàin　表面性の痛み

ténder pàin　触ったときの痛み

thróbbing pàin　拍動性の痛み，ズキズキする痛み

*Match the words with their opposites.*

1. sharp      2. acute      3. generalized

4. constant      5. severe      6. deep

7. sudden

chronic    localized    dull    mild    periodic    gradual    superficial

*Fill in the blanks.*

1. His _____ aches.
2. He has a mild rash on his _____ .
3. He has a stiff _____ .
4. His _____ hurts.
5. He has a cut on his _____ .
6. He has a tender pain on his _____ .
7. He feels a sharp pain in his _____ .
8. His _____ hurts.
9. He is complaining of a dull pain in his _____ .
10. He has a prickly pain in his _____ .

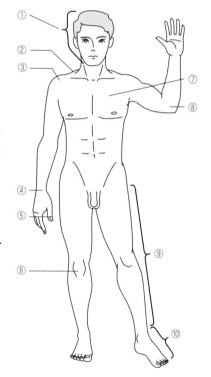

physician 医師

internist, physician 内科医

surgeon 外科医

resident 研修医

attending physician, doctor in charge 担当医

dentist 歯科医師

nurse 看護師

associate nurse, assistant nurse 准看護師

nursing assistant, nurse's aide 看護助手

midwife 助産師

pharmacist 薬剤師

occupational therapist [OT] 作業療法士

physical therapist [PT] 理学療法士

speech-language-hearing therapist [ST] 言語聴覚士

medical social worker [MSW] 医療ソーシャルワーカー

psychiatric social worker [PSW] 精神保健福祉士

dietician, nutritionist 栄養士

laboratory technician 検査技師

clerk 事務職員

receptionist 受付事務(職員)

paramedic, emergency medical technician [EMT] 救急救命士

medical interpreter 医療通訳

janitor 用務員

guard 警備員

cleaner, cleaning staff, cleaning man [woman] 清掃員

volunteer ボランティア

# Chapter 6 — Daily Activities

## Let's Listen

*Nurse Yuta Sanada is getting some information from his patient, Mrs. Martin, about her daily activities.*

| | |
|---|---|
| **Nurse** | Hello, Mrs. Martin. How are you doing? |
| **Mrs. Martin** | Fine. |
| **Nurse** | I'd like to ask you about some of your daily activities. |
| **Mrs. Martin** | OK. |
| **Nurse** | How many hours do you usually sleep at night? |
| **Mrs. Martin** | Oh, I guess about eight and a half hours. |
| **Nurse** | Do you ever have any difficulty sleeping? |
| **Mrs. Martin** | Hardly ever. |
| **Nurse** | How many meals do you eat a day? |
| **Mrs. Martin** | Usually three, but sometimes I skip lunch. |
| **Nurse** | How's your appetite? |
| **Mrs. Martin** | Not very good. I don't feel like eating. |
| **Nurse** | Any difficulty with your bowel movements? |
| **Mrs. Martin** | No, I'm very regular. |
| **Nurse** | Do you usually do any exercise? |
| **Mrs. Martin** | I try to swim at the gym when I have time. |

1. dáily actívities     2. swállow     3. líquid     4. irrégular

5. occásionally     6. fréquently     7. álcohol     8. aeróbics

9. recreátional drúg

10. I'd like to ask you about some of your daily activities.

11. How many hours do you usually sleep at night?

12. How many meals do you eat a day?

13. Do you have any difficulty with your bowel movements?

14. Do you smoke?

15. How often do you drink alcohol?

16. What kind of exercise do you get?

## NOTES

生活習慣について尋ねる項目

通例，睡眠と休息，食習慣，排泄，喫煙・飲酒，運動などを尋ねる．このほか，米国のナースは recreational drugs*や social support**/family support について次のような質問をする．

Do you ever use any recreational drugs?

How often do you get a chance to meet and talk about your problems with a family member or a friend?

---

\* recreational drugs：快楽用麻薬（治療用麻薬に対して）．

\*\* social support：周囲の人から与えられる物理的・心理的支援．

37

*Ask your partner about some of her/his daily activities. Fill out the chart below. After you have finished, exchange roles with her/him.*

Conversation starter : I'd like to ask you about some of your daily activities.

Name : _____

(your partner's name)

1. Hours of Sleep : She/He sleeps (        ) hours.
   ☐ 8  ☐ 7  ☐ 6  ☐ seven and a half  ☐ _____

2. Meals : She/He eats (        ) meals a day.
   ☐ three  ☐ two

   She/He skips (        ).
   ☐ breakfast  ☐ lunch  ☐ dinner

3. Appetite : ☐ Her/His appetite has been good.
   ☐ She/He doesn't have much appetite.
   ☐ She/He has no appetite.
   ☐ She/He can't swallow anything but liquids.

4. Bowel Movements : ☐ Her/His bowel movements are regular.
   ☐ Her/His bowel movements are irregular.
   ☐ She/He is/has been constipated for (        ) day(s).

5. Smoking : ☐ She/He smokes often.  ☐ She/He smokes occasionally.
   ☐ She/He seldom smokes.  ☐ She/He never smokes.

6. Drinking : ☐ She/He drinks alcohol often.
   ☐ She/He drinks alcohol occasionally.
   ☐ She/He seldom drinks alcohol.
   ☐ She/He never drinks alcohol.

7. Recreational drugs : She/He (        ) uses recreational drugs.
   ☐ frequently  ☐ socially
   ☐ occasionally  ☐ rarely or never

8. Exercise：She/He (☐ regularly ☐ sometimes ) _____.
   ☐ swims         ☐ jogs          ☐ takes a walk
   ☐ does aerobics  ☐ plays tennis   ☐ _____.

9. Hobbies：She/He has _____.
   ☐ one or more hobbies   ☐ no hobbies
   She/He likes to _____.
   ☐ play the piano   ☐ cook   ☐ play online games
   ☐ _____

10. Social/Family Support：She/He has _____.
    ☐ frequent contact with friends/relatives
    ☐ occasional contact with friends/relatives
    ☐ little or no contact with friends/relatives

11. Any other information：_____.
    (Speak freely.)
    (e.g. She/He's a vegetarian./She/He prefers Western food./She/He often
    works till late at night.)

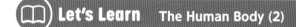
Head (頭部)

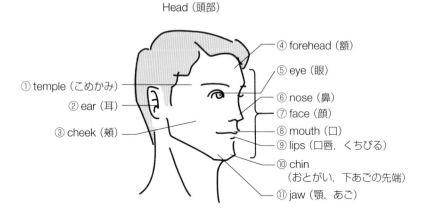

④ forehead (額)

⑤ eye (眼)

① temple (こめかみ)

② ear (耳)

⑥ nose (鼻)

⑦ face (顔)

③ cheek (頬)

⑧ mouth (口)

⑨ lips (口唇, くちびる)

⑩ chin
(おとがい, 下あごの先端)

⑪ jaw (顎, あご)

Torso & Arm (体幹と腕)

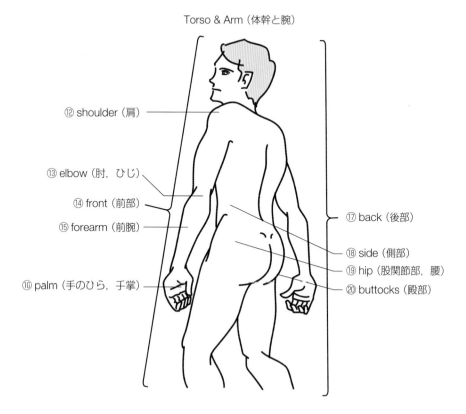

⑫ shoulder (肩)

⑬ elbow (肘, ひじ)

⑭ front (前部)

⑰ back (後部)

⑮ forearm (前腕)

⑱ side (側部)

⑲ hip (股関節部, 腰)

⑩ palm (手のひら, 手掌)

⑳ buttocks (殿部)

*Fill in the blanks.*

Head（頭部）

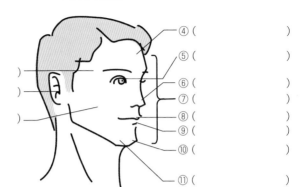

① ( 　　　　 )
② ( 　　　　 )
③ ( 　　　　 )

④ ( 　　　　　　　　 )
⑤ ( 　　　　　　　　 )
⑥ ( 　　　　　　　　 )
⑦ ( 　　　　　　　　 )
⑧ ( 　　　　　　　　 )
⑨ ( 　　　　　　　　 )
⑩ ( 　　　　　　　　 )
⑪ ( 　　　　　　　　 )

Torso & Arm（体幹と腕）

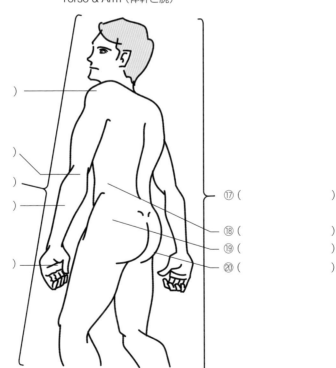

⑫ ( 　　　　 )
⑬ ( 　　　　 )
⑭ ( 　　　　 )
⑮ ( 　　　　 )
⑯ ( 　　　　 )

⑰ ( 　　　　　　　　 )
⑱ ( 　　　　　　　　 )
⑲ ( 　　　　　　　　 )
⑳ ( 　　　　　　　　 )

*The Health Questionnaire*     *Answer YES or NO.*

1. Do you maintain your weight within normal limits?     YES ☐   NO ☐

2. Do you eat three meals each day?     YES ☐   NO ☐

3. Do you have regular bowel movements?     YES ☐   NO ☐

4. Do you get at least seven hours of sleep each night?     YES ☐   NO ☐

5. Do you usually sleep soundly and wake up feeling
   energetic in the morning?     YES ☐   NO ☐

6. Do you engage in physical activities each day?     YES ☐   NO ☐

7. Are you a nonsmoker?     YES ☐   NO ☐

8. Do you drink alcohol in moderation?     YES ☐   NO ☐

9. Do you wear seat belts in the car?     YES ☐   NO ☐

10. Do you have close friends?     YES ☐   NO ☐

11. Are you living your everyday life fully?     YES ☐   NO ☐

12. Do you have regular health checkups?     YES ☐   NO ☐

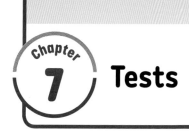

# Tests

## Chapter 7

## Let's Listen

*Nurse Seki is going to do several lab tests.*

**Nurse**   Please tell me your name and date of birth.

**Ms. Russo**   OK. My name is Maria Russo, and I was born on December 12, 1995.

**Nurse**   Thank you.

**Ms. Russo**   Do I need to do anything?

**Nurse**   Yes, we need a sample of your urine. Please use this cup to collect your mid-stream urine. First, urinate a small amount into the toilet. Then a small amount into the cup − about one-third. After that, leave the cup on the rack in the toilet.

**Ms. Russo**   I understand.

(a little later)

**Nurse**   Now, we need a blood sample. Sit here, please. Relax your arm. Is it all right if I use alcohol wipes?

**Ms. Russo**   Sure, no problem.

**Nurse**   I'll put this tourniquet around your arm. It'll feel tight. Please make a tight fist, like this. Good. There'll be a little prick. Ready?

**Ms. Russo**   Are you finished? That wasn't too bad.

1. láb tèsts　　2. míd-stream úrine　　3. úrinate　　4. blóod sàmple

5. álcohol wìpes　　6. tóurniquet　　7. màke a físt　　8. X́-ray depàrtment

9. inflammátion　　10. ántigen

11. Úrinate a small amóunt into the toilet.

12. Is it all ríght if I use álcohol wipes?

13. I'll put this tóurniquet around your árm.

14. You must nót eat or drínk anything.

1. 〜しなければならない

There're several lab tests that we *must* do.

いくつか検査をしなければなりません.

❶ must は義務・強制・必要を表す.

What do I *have to* do?　何をしなければなりませんか.

❶ have to ... はより口語的な表現.

2. 〜してはいけない (禁止)

You *must not* eat or drink anything.　飲食物は何もとってはいけません.

❶ must not は強い禁止を表す.　may not, can't [cannot] は must not [mustn't] より弱く, 口語的.　shouldn't は「〜しないほうがよい」というニュアンスで使う.

3. 〜してもよいか (許可を求める)

*Could* [*Can*] I have any water?　水をいただけますか, 水が飲めますか.

No, I'm afraid you *can't*.　いいえ, 飲めません. だめです.

*May* I get out of bed?　ベッドを離れてもよいでしょうか.

No, you *must not*.　いいえ, 絶対いけません.

❶ Could I ... は, 〜してもよいかと許可を求める丁寧な表現.　May I ... はやや格式ばった丁寧な言い方.　Can I ... はやや砕けた口語的表現.

*Is it all right if I* take away the tray?　トレーを片付けてもよろしいでしょうか.

❶ Is it all right if I ... も, 丁寧な尋ね方.

44

# 💬 Let's Speak

*Arrange these directions in the proper order by numbering the statements. Then, explain the procedures to your partner. Use the following expressions for a nurse, while your partner is using the ones for a patient. Your partner should close her/his textbook while you are speaking. After you have finished, exchange roles with her/him.*

[a nurse]  We need _____ ./We'd like to take your _____.
First,/Then,/After that, _____ , (please)./I'll _____.
You must _____ ./You must not _____./Don't _____.
Is it all right if I _____?/(Are you) Ready?

[a patient]  OK./I understand./Sure. No problem./Do I need to do anything?/
Finished?

1. Urine sample : ( to collect your mid-stream urine)
   __ leave the cup on the rack in the toilet
   __ fill about one-third of the cup
   __ urinate a small amount into the toilet

2. Blood sample :
   __ use alcohol wipes
   __ relax your arm
   __ make a fist
   __ put this tourniquet around your arm

3. Stomach X-ray :
   __ eat supper the night before the test
   __ go to the X-ray department
   __ not eat or drink anything after midnight

4. TB test :
   __ look for signs for inflammation
   __ come back here in two days
   __ inject a small amount of antigen under your skin

INTERNAL（内部）

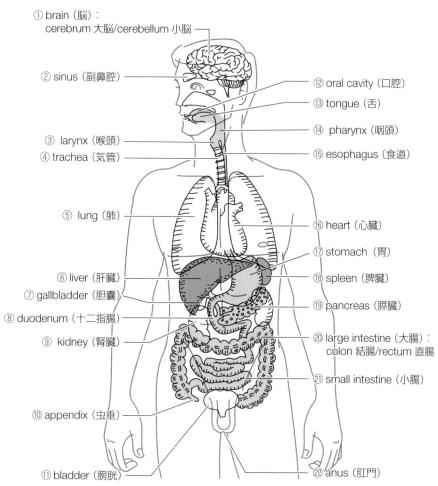

① brain（脳）：
    cerebrum 大脳/cerebellum 小脳

② sinus（副鼻腔）

③ larynx（喉頭）
④ trachea（気管）

⑤ lung（肺）

⑥ liver（肝臓）
⑦ gallbladder（胆嚢）
⑧ duodenum（十二指腸）
⑨ kidney（腎臓）

⑩ appendix（虫垂）

⑪ bladder（膀胱）

⑫ oral cavity（口腔）
⑬ tongue（舌）
⑭ pharynx（咽頭）
⑮ esophagus（食道）

⑯ heart（心臓）
⑰ stomach（胃）
⑱ spleen（脾臓）
⑲ pancreas（膵臓）
⑳ large intestine（大腸）：
    colon 結腸/rectum 直腸
㉑ small intestine（小腸）

㉒ anus（肛門）

*Fill in the blanks.*

INTERNAL （内部）

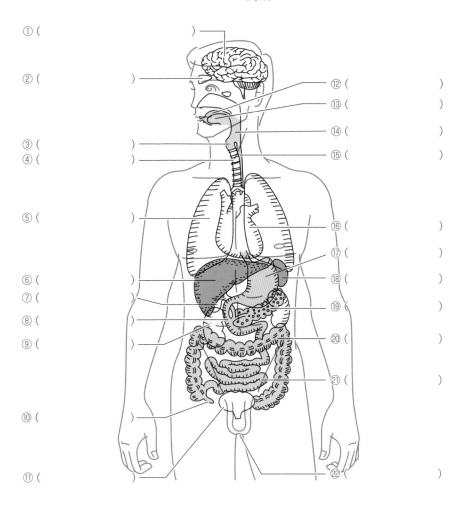

① (                    )

② (                    )                                    ⑫ (                    )
                                                            ⑬ (                    )
                                                            ⑭ (                    )
③ (                    )                                    ⑮ (                    )
④ (                    )

⑤ (                    )                                    ⑯ (                    )
                                                            ⑰ (                    )
⑥ (                    )                                    ⑱ (                    )
⑦ (                    )
⑧ (                    )                                    ⑲ (                    )
⑨ (                    )
                                                            ⑳ (                    )

                                                            ㉑ (                    )

⑩ (                    )

⑪ (                    )                                    ㉒ (                    )

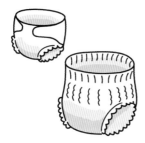

diaper（幼児用おむつ）
adult［incontinence］briefs*（成人用おむつ）

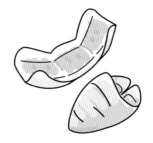

incontinence pad（失禁パッド）

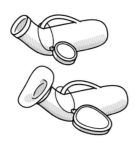

urinal bottle（尿器，しびん）

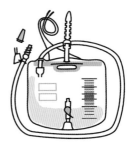

urine（collection）bag（採尿バッグ）

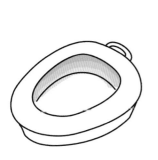

bedpan（ベッド用便器）

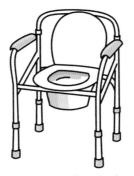

commode（椅子便器）

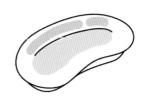

kidney basin（膿盆）

---

\* adult diaper も用いられるが，不愉快に思う患者がいるので避けたい．

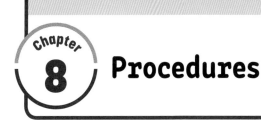

# Procedures

Let's Listen

**A** *Mr. Ling had surgery yesterday. Nurse Hara is making medication rounds.*

| | |
|---|---|
| **Nurse** | Mr. Ling, the doctor has ordered an injection for your pain. You may have it every four hours if you need it. Would you like it now? |
| **Mr. Ling** | Yes, please. I hurt so much. |
| **Nurse** | OK. There'll be a little prick. Here it is …. Does your IV site hurt? |
| **Mr. Ling** | No, I don't notice it. |
| **Nurse** | Good. The pain will go away after a while. Now, I have a couple of pills for you to swallow. |
| **Mr. Ling** | OK. |

..........................................................................

**B** *Some time later Nurse Hara has changed Mr. Ling's dressing.*

| | |
|---|---|
| **Nurse** | Mr. Ling, it's all finished. You are healing nicely, and you have a fresh bandage. |
| **Mr. Ling** | Thank you. |
| **Nurse** | Now it's time for you to rest. |
| **Mr. Ling** | OK. |

1. procédures   2. injéction   3. a còuple of pílls   4. dréssing chànge

5. béd rèst   6. lów sált dìet   7. déep bréathing èxercise   8. féed

9. exáctly as dirécted

10. Now it's time for you to rest.

11. The doctor has ordered bed rest.


## NOTES

1. 頻度の表現

（1）～ごと，～おき

The doctor has ordered an injection for your pain. You may have it every four hours.

先生から痛み止めを注射するようにとの指示がありました．4時間あければいいですよ．

every two hours   2時間ごと，every three days   3日おき

（2）（ある期間に）何回，何度

once a day   1日に1回，two times（twice）a day   1日に2回

❶3回以上は ... times を使う．

❶a day の代わりに per day とも言う．

three times per day   1日3回，60 drops per minute   毎分60滴

2.（人が）～をする時間であることを促す表現

It's time for you to rest.／It's time for your rest.   休息の時間ですよ．

"It's time for *somebody* to do ...." は，(誰かが)～をする時間であることを知らせ促す意味を表す．

*Imagine that you are going to remind your patient to do something. As your partner says the words on the left, you say the sentences on the right. While you are speaking, close your textbook. Exchange roles with her/him.*

| Your partner | You |
|---|---|
| 1. The doctor has ordered bed rest.<br>an injection for your pain<br>a low salt diet<br>deep breathing exercises<br>a dressing change | a) The doctor has ordered bed rest.<br>b)<br>c)<br>d)<br>e) |
| 2. Now, it's time for you to rest.<br>take your medication<br>have a bed bath<br>go to the X-ray department<br>feed your baby | a) Now, it's time for you to rest.<br>b)<br>c)<br>d)<br>e) |
| 3. Please take this medication every four hours.<br>when you get up<br>with a lot of water<br>when you can't sleep<br>exactly as directed | a) Please take this medication every four hours.<br>b)<br>c)<br>d)<br>e) |
| 4. I have a couple of pills for you to swallow.<br>a hospital gown for you to wear<br>another pillow for you to put between your knees<br>a booklet about a low salt diet for you to read | a) I have a couple of pills for you to swallow.<br>b)<br>c)<br>d) |

Urogenital Organs（泌尿生殖器）

female（女性）

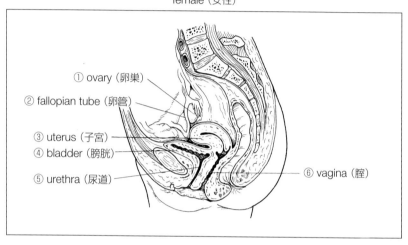

① ovary（卵巣）

② fallopian tube（卵管）

③ uterus（子宮）

④ bladder（膀胱）

⑤ urethra（尿道）

⑥ vagina（腟）

male（男性）

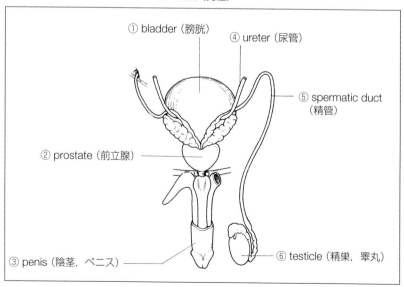

① bladder（膀胱）

④ ureter（尿管）

⑤ spermatic duct（精管）

② prostate（前立腺）

③ penis（陰茎，ペニス）

⑥ testicle（精巣，睾丸）

*Fill in the blanks.*

Urogenital Organs（泌尿生殖器）

female（女性）

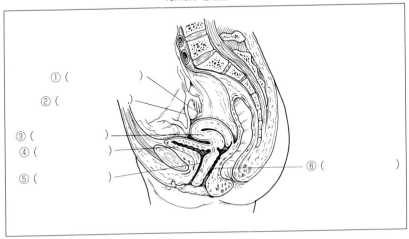

① (　　　　　　　)
② (　　　　　　　)
③ (　　　　　　　)
④ (　　　　　　　)
⑤ (　　　　　　　)
⑥ (　　　　　　　　　　)

male（男性）

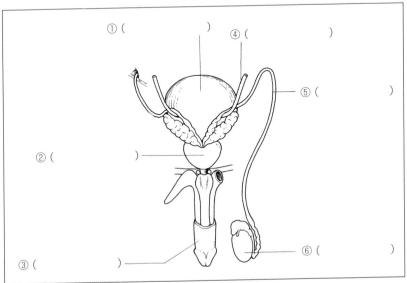

① (　　　　　　　)
② (　　　　　　　)
③ (　　　　　　　)
④ (　　　　　　　　)
⑤ (　　　　　　　　)
⑥ (　　　　　　　　)

## 1. Pursed-lip breathing（口すぼめ呼吸）

With your mouth shut, please breathe through your nose normally.

Purse your lips as if you're whistling.

Breathe out slowly through your pursed lips.

Be careful not to push yourself too hard to force the air out.

Breathe out twice as slowly as you breathed in.

After some practice try to gradually increase the time to breathe out ［make breathing out longer］ and slow ［reduce］ your breathing rate.

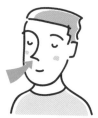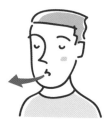

## 2. Abdominal breathing（腹式呼吸）

First, please lie on your back.

Relax, and place your hand（s）on your abdomen.

Breathe in slowly through your nose.

Try to feel that your abdomen gets larger as you breathe in.

Breathe out slowly through your pursed lips.

Try to feel that your abdomen falls inward as you breathe out.

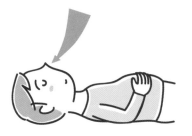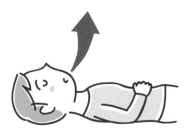

# Positioning the Patient in Bed

 **Let's Listen**

*Nurse Naka is positioning Mr. Smith in bed after surgery.*

**Nurse**  Mr. Smith, you need to change your position often so that you won't get a bedsore or pneumonia.

**Mr. Smith**  It hurts so much. I don't feel like turning at all.

**Nurse**  I know. I'll help you change your position.

**Mr. Smith**  Please do it gently so that I don't feel any pain.

**Nurse**  OK. Now you're going to turn to your right. First, move your left arm over to your right. Now, bend your left knee and cross it over to the right.

**Mr. Smith**  Like this?

**Nurse**  Good. Let me straighten your sheets. Could you roll over to one side, please?

**Mr. Smith**  That feels much better.

**Nurse**  I'm going to put a pillow under your left leg and another one behind your back.

**Mr. Smith**  Thank you. I'm much more comfortable now.

1. bédsore     2. pneumónia     3. posítion     4. túrn to your ríght

5. túrn to your léft     6. bénd your knées     7. stráighten

8. róll òver to òne síde     9. cómfortable     10. píllowcase     11. flúff

12. táke this snáck tràry awáy     13. líe down on your báck

14. sít on the édge of your béd

15. I'll hélp you chánge your posítion.

1. 援助 (assistance) を申し出る場合

   I'll help you change your position.

   体の向きを変えるのをお手伝いしましょう.

   ❶ 米語では, help のあとには通例 to をつけない.

2. 命令 (command) する場合

   Bend your knees.   膝を曲げてください.

   (否定形) Don't bend your knees.   膝を曲げないで.

   ❶ イントネーションにより「〜するな」に相当する強い語調となる.

3. 依頼 (request) する場合

   Please open your mouth.   どうぞ口を開けてください.

   Roll up your sleeve, please.   どうぞ袖をまくり上げてください.

   (丁寧な形)

   Could you make a fist?   握りこぶしをつくっていただけますか.

   Could you please turn over?   反対向きになっていただけませんか.

   (否定形) Please don't move.   どうぞ動かないでください.

4. 「〜するように」という目的を表す表現   so that ...

   You need to change your position frequently so that you won't/will not get a bedsore or pneumonia.   褥瘡(床ずれ)や肺炎を起こさないように頻繁に体位を変えなくてはいけません.

   ❶ so that ... に続く動詞は can, may, will などの助動詞を伴うことが多い.

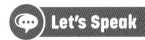 

*As your partner says the words on the left, you say the sentences on the right.*
*While you are speaking, close your textbook. Exchange roles with her/him.*

| Your partner | You |
|---|---|
| 1. I'm going to change your bed sheets.<br>change the pillowcase<br>take this snack tray away<br>make you a little more comfortable<br>put a pillow behind your back | a) I'm going to change your bed sheets.<br>b)<br>c)<br>d)<br>e) |
| 2. Let me straighten your sheets.<br>fluff your pillow<br>turn off the light<br>bring another blanket<br>raise your bed | a) Let me straighten your sheets.<br>b)<br>c)<br>d)<br>e) |
| 3. I'll help you change your position.<br>take a bath<br>go to the restroom<br>brush your teeth<br>sit in your wheelchair | a) I'll help you change your position.<br>b)<br>c)<br>d)<br>e) |
| 4. Could you roll over to one side?<br>turn to your right<br>bend your knees<br>lie down on your back<br>sit on the edge of your bed | a) Could you roll over to one side?<br>b)<br>c)<br>d)<br>e) |

Common Illnesses and Conditions

állergy　アレルギー
　❶ 通例，複数形 allergies を用いる.

angína　狭心症

arthrítis　関節炎

ásthma　喘息

áthlete's fóot　足白癬

bronchítis　気管支炎

cáncer　がん

cátaract　白内障

chícken pòx　水痘

cómmon cóld　感冒

constipátion　便秘

cystítis　膀胱炎

depréssion　うつ病

diabétes　糖尿病
　❶ type 1 と type 2 がある.

diarrhéa　下痢

dislocátion　脱臼

eczéma　湿疹

emphyséma　（肺）気腫

frácture　骨折

gàstroenterítis　胃腸炎

háy fèver　花粉症

héart attàck　心臓発作
　❶ myocárdial infárction（心筋梗塞）
　とも言う.

hígh blóod prèssure　高血圧（症）
　❶ hyperténsion とも言う.

influénza［flú］
　インフルエンザ，流行性感冒

màlnutrítion　栄養失調

méasles　麻疹

míddle éar infèction　中耳炎
　❶ otítis média とも言う.

múmps　流行性耳下腺炎

obésity　肥満

pharyngítis　咽頭炎
　❶ sóre thróat とも言う.

pneumónia　肺炎

pòsttraumátic stréss disòrder［PTSD］
　心的外傷後ストレス障害

rubélla　風疹
　❶ Gérman méasles とも言う.

séxually transmítted infèction
　［STI］　性感染症

shíngles　帯状疱疹
　❶ hérpes zóster とも言う.

stróke　脳卒中

tuberculósis［TB］　結核

*Fill in the blanks with appropriate terms.*

1. Dust and pollen make Mrs. Kato sneeze. She has _____ to them.
2. Many people on the subway wear masks during the changes of seasons. They have _____ .
3. Mr. Seto ate a very spicy meal last night. Later he experienced many loose bowel movements or loose stools. The doctor said he has _____ .
4. The nurse explained to a group of college girls that if they severely restricted their calorie intake without paying attention to proper nutrients, they might develop severe _____ .
5. The baby was pulling on his left ear and screaming. His mother suspected that he had _____ .
6. In Japan there are many snacks and fast foods available now. The incidence of _____ is rising.
7. When people who smoke heavily develop a great difficulty in exhaling [breathing out], they are showing a symptom of _____ .
8. Mr. Thompson needs to give himself an insulin injection every day, because he has _____ .

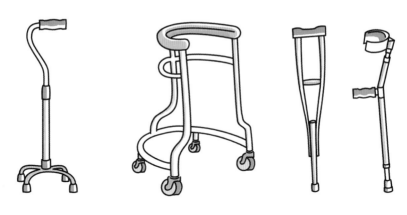

quad cane（四脚杖）　　　　walker（歩行器）　　　　crutches（松葉杖）

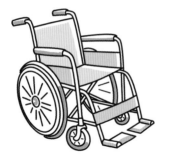
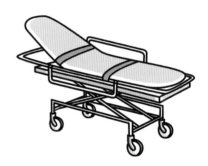

wheelchair（車椅子）　　　　　　　gurney（車輪付き担架）

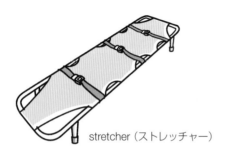
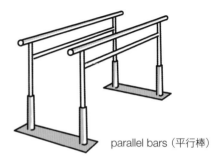

stretcher（ストレッチャー）　　　parallel bars（平行棒）

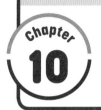

# Chapter 10 Bath and Comfort

*Nurse Tani is giving Mrs. Olson a bed bath now.*

**Nurse**  I'm going to give you a bed bath now.

**Mrs. Olson**  Great. I've been wanting one. I feel so sweaty and my skin is oily.

**Nurse**  Would you like a shampoo?

**Mrs. Olson**  Not yet. I hurt too much.

**Nurse**  OK. First I'll do your face and neck. … Now your arms and chest. Could you turn to the side?

**Mrs. Olson**  Sure.

**Nurse**  I'll wash your back and rub it with lotion.

**Mrs. Olson**  That's so relaxing.

**Nurse**  Good. Now, your legs and feet. There … can you reach down to wash your private area?

**Mrs. Olson**  Yes, I think so.

**Nurse**  OK. I'll just step behind the curtain. Let me know if you need any help.

(a little later)

**Mrs. Olson**  I do feel refreshed, thank you.

1. béd bàth    2. shampóo    3. báck rùb    4. hàve anóther blánket

5. brúsh your téeth    6. tàke sléeping pìlls

7. hàve an injéction to éase your pain    8. tàke a wálk to the lóunge

9. Let me know if you need any help.

10. Would you like a back rub?

11. Would you like to have a back rub?

12. Yes, please.    13. No, thank you.

14. Then, tell us when you feel like having a bed bath.

1. 相手の意向を尋ねる丁寧な表現

   Would you like a shampoo?　シャンプーをいたしましょうか.

   Would you like to drink some water?　お水が飲みたくありませんか.

   ❶ Do you want/like to drink ...?　（飲みたいですか）よりも婉曲的で丁寧な表現.

2. 意向を聞かれた場合の応答

   （肯定）Yes, please.　ええ, お願いします.

   　　　　Yes, I'd like to.　はい, そうしたいです.

   （否定）No, thank you.　いいえ, けっこうです.

   　　　　No, not now.　今はけっこうです.

3. 気分を尋ねる

   How do you feel?　ご気分はいかがですか.

   I feel ....　... の部分に形容詞を使っていろいろの感覚が表現できる.

   〔例〕I feel dizzy.　めまいがする. I feel chilly.　寒気がする.

   　　　I feel cold.　寒い. I feel fatigued.　疲労感がある.

   　　　I feel feverish.　熱っぽい. I feel refreshed.　さっぱりした.

*Imagine that you have been in the hospital for more than two weeks. Read through the following phrases and put checks in the boxes you'd like to do. Then, have a conversation with your partner using the expressions in the examples below. While you are asking, your partner should try to close her/ his textbook. After you have finished, exchange roles with her/him.*

（Example）

Nurse：Would you like something to eat?

Would you like to have something to eat?

Patient：Oh, Yes, please. I'm so hungry.　　No, thank you. I have no appetite.

Yes, I'd like to.　　　　　　　No, not now. I'm not hungry.

Nurse：Then, I'll bring _____ right away.　OK. Then, tell us when you feel

like _____ ing.

（Nurse 参考例）I'll be glad to help you.／I'll help you do it.／I'll go with you.

OK. Tell us when you need it（them）.／Let us know when you

want to _____.／OK. Is there anything else I can do for you?

|  | Yes No |  | Yes No |
|---|---|---|---|
| 1. a back rub | ☐ ☐ | 2. some water | ☐ ☐ |
| 3. another blanket | ☐ ☐ | 4. have a shampoo | ☐ ☐ |
| 5. have a bed bath | ☐ ☐ | 6. brush your teeth | ☐ ☐ |
| 7. walk to the bathroom | ☐ ☐ | 8. read newspapers | ☐ ☐ |
| 9. do deep breathing exercises | ☐ ☐ | 10. take sleeping pills | ☐ ☐ |
| 11. have an injection to ease your pain | ☐ ☐ | | |
| 12. take a walk to the lounge | ☐ ☐ | | |

## Prefixes (1)

a-, an- 否定［無，不，非］     *á*pathy 無感動，無関心   *á*pnea 無呼吸   *an*émia 貧血

ab- はずれた，それた     *ab*nórmal 異常の   *ab*dúction 外転

ante- 前の，前方の     *ant*érior 前方の   *ante*merídian 午前の

anti- 抗，反，対     *anti*biótics 抗菌薬，抗生物質   *anti*tóxin 抗毒素

bi- 二，重，双，複     *bi*fócal 二焦点性の   *bi*língual バイリンガルの

bi(o)- 生物の，生命の     *bi*ólogy 生物学   *bi*opsy 生検

cardi(o)- 心臓の     *cardi*ólogist 循環器内科医   *cardio*mégaly 心肥大

co-, com-, con- 共同，共通，相互     *có*lleague 同僚，仲間   *com*plicátion 合併症   *con*grúity 適合，一致

contra- 反対，逆，抗     *contra*céption 避妊

dec(a)- 10，10 倍を表す     *déc*ade 10 年間

dys- 痛みのある，悪い，困難な     *dýs*pnea 呼吸困難   *dys*fúnction 機能不全

end(o)- 中へ，内部の     *éndo*crine 内分泌の，内分泌腺   *éndo*scòpe 内視鏡

equi- 等しい     *equi*líbrium 平衡   *equi*valent 同量の，等価の

eu- よい，やさしい     *eu*pépsia 消化良好   *eu*phória 多幸（症）   *eu*thanásia 安楽死

ex(o)- 外へ，外から，外部の     *ex*hále （息などを）吐く   *ex*ótic 外来性の

extra- 外の，超の     *extra*céllular 細胞外の   *extra*váscular 脈管外の   *extra*sénsory 超感覚的な

gastr(o)- 胃の     *gástro*scope 胃内視鏡   *gastr*ítis 胃炎

gynec(o)- 女性の     *gynec*ólogy 婦人科（学）   *gynec*ólogist 婦人科医

hem(o)-, hema- 血の     *hemo*glóbin ヘモグロビン   *hémo*rrhoids

|  |  |
|---|---|
|  | 痔　*hemo*phília　血友病 |
| hemi- 半分の | *hémi*sphere（大脳，小脳の）半球　*hemi*plégia 片麻痺 |
| hepat(o)- 肝臓の | *hepat*ítis　肝炎　*hepát*ic cirrhósis　肝硬変 |
| homo-, homeo- 同一の | *homó*genous　同種の，均質の　*homeo*stásis 恒常性［ホメオスタシス］　*homo*séxual　同性愛の |
| hyper- より高い，過度の | *hyper*ténsion　高血圧　*hyper*thýroidism　甲状腺機能亢進（症） |
| hypo- より低い，低度の | *hypo*ténsion　低血圧　*hypo*glycémia　低血糖（症） |
| idio- 個別的な，特異的な | *idio*páthic　特発（性）の　*idio*sýncrasy　特異体質 |
| inter- 間の | *inter*míttent　間欠性の　*inter*áction　相互作用 |
| intra-, intro- 内部の | *intra*váscular　血管内の　*intra*vénous drìp ［IV drìp］点滴　*intro*vérsion　内向，内転 |
| later(o)- 片側の | *láter*al　側面の，片側の，外側の *latero*posítion　側位，側方転位 ❶片側にずれていること． |
| leuk(o)- 白い | *léuko*cyte　白血球　*leuk*émia　白血病 |
| mal- 悪い，不良な | *mal*fúnction　機能不全　*mal*nutrítion　栄養不良 |
| mon(o)- 単一の | *mono*chromátic　単色の，一色の　*mon*ócular 一眼性の |
| multi- 多数の，多産の | *múlti*form　多形の　*múlti*ple chóice　多肢選択の |
| my(o)- 筋の，筋肉の | *myo*cárdium　心筋　*myó*ma　筋腫 |
| neo- 新しい | *néo*nate　新生児　*neo*plásm　新生物，腫瘍 |
| nephr(o)- 腎臓の | *nephr*ítis　腎炎　*nephr*éctomy　腎摘除 |
| neur(o)- 神経の | *neur*ítis　神経炎　*neur*ólogist　神経内科医 |

Find in [Column 2] the matching definition of the term given in [Column 1].

| [Column 1] | [Column 2] |
|---|---|
| 1. euphoria | a. decrease in hemoglobin in the blood |
| 2. dysfunction | b. an optical instrument for the visualization of the interior of an organ of the body |
| 3. anemia | c. drawing away from the midline |
| 4. complication | d. breathe out |
| 5. endoscope | e. a feeling or state of well-being or elation |
| 6. antitoxin | f. before noon, morning |
| 7. abduction | g. a process or technique for prevention of pregnancy |
| 8. exhale | h. a secondary disease occurring during a primary disease or condition |
| 9. contraception | i. opposing the action of a poison |
| 10. antemeridian | j. being unable to function normally |

Draw a vertical line to separate the prefix from the rest of the term. Then write the definition of the prefix after the term.

| | | |
|---|---|---|
| 1. idiosyncrasy | 2. neoplasm | 3. intermittent |
| 4. intravascular | 5. hypertension | 6. lateroposition |
| 7. gastritis | 8. hemoglobin | 9. malnutrition |
| 10. hypotension | 11. hemiplegia | 12. homogenous |
| 13. monocular | 14. multiform | 15. leukemia |

① It'll be all right.／You'll be all right.　大丈夫ですよ.

② Please relax.　どうぞ楽にしてください.

③ It'll be over in a few minutes.　2〜3 分で済みますよ.

④ Don't worry.　ご心配いりません.

⑤ We'll take care of everything.　私どもがすべてお世話いたします.

⑥ I'll stay with you.　私がそばについています.

⑦ Hold my hand.　私の手を握ってください.

⑧ You'll feel better soon.　すぐに楽になりますよ.

⑨ You're doing well.　調子はいいですよ.

⑩ Don't give up.　あきらめてはいけません.

⑪ You'll get better soon.／You'll soon be well again.

すぐによくなりますよ.

⑫ You did well.　よくがんばりましたね.

⑬ You've really had a hard time.　つらかったでしょう.

⑭ Your baby is doing well.　赤ちゃんは元気ですよ.

⑮ You'll be able to leave the hospital soon.／You can go home soon.

すぐに退院できますよ.

⑯ Take（good）care of yourself.／Take care!

（どうぞ）お大事に！

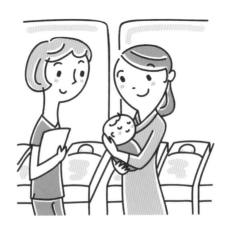

# Patient Teaching

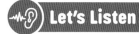
**A** *Nurse Kato is reviewing instructions from the doctor with Mr. Jones.*

**Nurse** Did you understand the doctor's instructions?

**Mr. Jones** Yes. I think she told me to take this medication, one tablet three times a day.

**Nurse** Do you remember whether to take it before or after meals?

**Mr. Jones** I'm not sure.

**Nurse** Before each meal is the best time. Do you recall what else she told you?

**Mr. Jones** She wants me to rest every afternoon.

**Nurse** Yes, that's right.

..............................................................................

**B** *Mrs. Payne has been diagnosed as having angina pectoris. Nurse Tajima has been instructing her about her medication and diet.*

**Nurse** You've had a lot to learn in the last few days. Let's review it.

**Mrs. Payne** Yes, that's a good idea.

**Nurse** Let's talk about your medication first. When did the doctor tell you to take it?

**Mrs. Payne** He said I should take the nitroglycerin whenever I feel chest pain.

**Nurse** Do you remember how to take nitroglycerin?

**Mrs. Payne** Oh, yes, I put it under my tongue and let it dissolve completely.

**Nurse** That's good. What else did he tell you?

**Mrs. Payne** He said I should cut down on salt and fatty foods.

**Nurse** What concerns you about the diet?

**Mrs. Payne** Well, it's not me that I'm concerned about. It's my family. I still have to cook for them and I'm not sure they will like it.

**Nurse** Actually, once you get into it, you'll find that your diet is a healthy one for the whole family.

**Mrs. Payne** We do like most of the foods on the diet. Only the way that we prepare the foods will change. No more frying.

1. táblet    2. nitroglýcerin    3. fátty fóod    4. fèel dízzy

5. fèel náuseated    6. a lòt of líquids    7. the óutpatient depàrtment

8. Let's review the doctor's instructions.

9. What else did he tell you?

10. What did the doctor tell you about your medication?

11. Do you remember when to take it?

12. He told me to take a good rest after meals.

13. Do you have any other questions?

薬の種類

oral medication  経口薬

   tablet  錠剤    pill  丸薬    liquid medication  水薬

   powder  散剤，粉薬    capsule  カプセル剤

external medication  外用薬  ❶ topical medication とも言う．

   suppository  坐薬    ointment  軟膏    poultice  湿布薬

inhalant  吸入薬

injection  注射薬

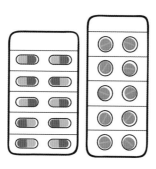

*Imagine that you are reviewing instructions from the doctor with your partner. Choose either (1), (2), or (3) and have some conversation, using the expressions below. You and your partner should not choose the same instructions. After you have finished, exchange roles with her/him.*

[You] Let's review the doctor's instructions.
What did he/she tell you about your medication/diet/exercise?
Do you remember how/when/what to _____?
What else did he/she tell you?
Yes, that's right./That's good./Exactly./Perfect./Anything else?
Do you have any other questions/concerns about it?

[Your partner] He/She told me to _____.
He/She said that I should _____.

(1) 1. Medication : take two tablets three times a day
　　　　　　　　　　 take them before each meal
　 2. Diet : cut down on salt and fatty foods
　 3. Others : get lots of rest
　　　　　　　　 call him/her if I/you feel dizzy or nauseated

(2) 1. Diet : eat plenty of fruits and vegetables, and low fat milk products
　　　　　　　 drink a lot of liquids
　 2. Exercise : get some light exercise
　 3. Others : take the medication every six hours
　　　　　　　　 come to the outpatient department next Friday, October 15

(3) 1. Exercise : exercise regularly
　　　　　　　　　 avoid hard exercise for a week
　 2. Medication : take it whenever I/you have the pain
　 3. Others : stop smoking
　　　　　　　　 check blood pressure periodically

(4) Speak freely.

## Prefixes (2)

non- 非, 不, 無                    *non*specífic　非特異性の　*non*atópic　非アトピー性の

oste(o)- 骨の                    *oste*álgia　骨痛　*osteo*porósis　骨粗鬆症

ophthalm(o)- 眼の                 *ophthalmó*logist　眼科医

rhin(o)- 鼻の                     *rhin*ítis　鼻炎　*rhino*pólyp　鼻ポリープ

path(o)- 疾病の                   *patho*génic　病因の　*pathó*logy　病理学

post- 後の, 後方の                *post*nátal　生後の　*post*óperative　術後(性)の

pre- 前の, 以前の                 *pre*medicátion　前投薬　*pre*nátal　出生前の

pseud(o)- 仮の, 偽りの             *pseudo*góut　偽痛風

psych(o)- 精神の, 心理の           *psych*íatry　精神医学　*psychó*logy　心理学

semi- 半分の                      *semi*cóma　半昏睡　*sèmi*sóft dìet　半流動食

sub- 下の, 下方の                 *sub*cónscious　意識下の, 潜在意識の
                                 *sub*cutáneous　皮下の

super- 上, 過, 超                 *super*ficial　外面の　*super*égo　超自我

sym-, syn- 合同, 結合, 合成        *sým*pathy　共感　*sýn*drome　症候群　*syn*thétic　合成の

ultra- 超                        *ultra*sound (test)　超音波検査　*ultra*víolet　紫外線

un- 無, 否                        *un*cónscious　無意識の　*un*éasy　不安な
                                 *un*restráined　無拘束の, 無制限の

uni- 単一の                       *uni*láteral　片側の, 一側の　*úni*sex　男女共通の

## Suffixes

-algia　痛み

myálgia　筋肉痛　neurálgia　神経痛

-cyte　細胞

lýmphocyte　リンパ球　erýthrocyte　赤血球

-ectomy　切除（術），摘出（術）

appendéctomy　虫垂切除（術）　tonsilléctomy
扁桃摘出（術）

-genic　生じる，発生する

cardiogénic　心臓性の，心臓に起因する
pathogénic　病因の

-glycemia　血糖（症）

hypoglycémia　低血糖（症）　hyperglycémia
高血糖（症）

-gram　図，記録，描くこと

electrocárdiogram［EKG/ECG］心電図
electroencéphalogram［EEG］脳波（図）

-graph, -graphy　描写装置，
図表，記録（法）

cárdiograph　心拍（動）記録器　tomógraphy
トモグラフィー，断層撮影（法）

-ism　状態，症状

áutism　自閉（症）　dwárfism　萎縮症，小人症

-itis　炎症

arthrítis　関節炎　sinusítis　静脈洞炎，副鼻
腔炎

-(o)logy　〜の研究，学

pathólogy　病理学　psychólogy　心理学

-oma　腫瘍

carcinóma　癌　hematóma　血腫　myóma
筋腫

-osis　異常増加，病的状態

alkalósis　アルカローシス　neurósis　神経症

-(o)stomy　開口部形成

colóstomy　人工肛門形成（術）　gastróstomy
胃ろう造設（術）

-pathy　苦痛，感情，疾患，療法

ápathy　無感動，無関心　neurópathy　神経
障害

-plasty　外科的修復

rhínoplasty　鼻形成（術）

-plegia　麻痺

hemiplégia　片麻痺　paraplégia　対麻痺

-scope, -scopy　検査器械，
検査（法）

stéthoscope　聴診器

-therapy　治療，療法

chèmothérapy　化学療法　psỳchothérapy
精神［心理］療法

73

EXERCISE 1

Put down the corresponding term in English.

1. 半流動食            2. 無意識の

3. 眼科医             4. 超自我

5. 関節炎             6. 生後の

7. 紫外線             8. 前投薬

9. 化学療法           10. 意識下の

11. 術後の            12. 病理学

EXERCISE 2

Find in the right column the matching definition of the suffix given in the left column, and write it in the space provided.

1. -(o)logy     _____ a. study of

2. -plegia      _____ b. instrument of examination

3. -oma         _____ c. creation of opening

4. -graph       _____ d. tumor

5. -algia       _____ e. condition

6. -cyte        _____ f. plastic surgery

7. -plasty      _____ g. pain

8. -ism         _____ h. excision

9. -scope       _____ i. cell

10. -ectomy     _____ j. something that is recorded or drawn

11. -therapy    _____ k. device for drawing

12. -(o)stomy   _____ l. inflammation

13. -genic      _____ m. producing

14. -gram       _____ n. paralysis

15. -itis       _____ o. medical treatment of disease by special means

- Be patient while your milk comes in.
- Sit comfortably with your back and arms supported when nursing.
- Clean your nipples with warm water and minimal soap.
- Alternate which side you start on.
- Burp your baby.
- Nurse frequently — whenever your baby wants.
- Drink a lot of liquids：water, tea, juice, and others.
- Get plenty of rest.
- Don't smoke.
- Don't drink alcohol.
- Ask your doctor if you should continue medications while breastfeeding.
- Don't be afraid to talk about your worries and seek out for help if you need it.

Enjoy your baby!

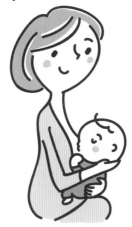

# Small Talk

## Let's Listen

**A** *Nurse Sato is working in Mr. Wade's room, and she takes time to chat with him about his family life.*

**Nurse**   Do you have a family with you here in Japan?

**Mr. Wade**   Yes – I am married and we have three kids, two boys and a girl.

**Nurse**   How old are your children?

**Mr. Wade**   Our sons are 8 and 10, and our daughter is 5.

**Nurse**   Tell me about your family of origin.

**Mr. Wade**   I have a brother who is older than me. My parents are still living in Ohio, and he lives near them with his family.

**Nurse**   Have they had a chance to visit you here in Japan?

**Mr. Wade**   Yes – my parents came last fall for three weeks, and my brother and his wife and kids are planning to visit next summer when school is out. And my wife's parents came for Christmas.

**Nurse**   That is wonderful. It must be hard to be separated from them.

**Mr. Wade**   Yes, but we Skype frequently so that our kids stay connected with their grandparents and cousins.

**B** *Nurse Sano is working in Mrs. Brown's room and she takes time to learn more about Mrs. Brown as a person and her experience with Japanese food.*

|  |  |
|---|---|
| **Nurse** | Where are you from? |
| **Mrs. Brown** | I'm from America. |
| **Nurse** | Oh, I once stayed in Los Angeles as an exchange student. My friends and host family were so friendly and kind. I really enjoyed American life. |
| **Mrs. Brown** | It's good to hear that you had a wonderful experience in my country. |
| **Nurse** | Speaking of America, which part of America are you from? |
| **Mrs. Brown** | I'm from Kentucky. |
| **Nurse** | Oh, Kentucky …, I love fried chicken. What's your favorite Japanese food? |
| **Mrs. Brown** | I love teriyaki-chicken, and sushi. |
| **Nurse** | Do your children eat sushi? |
| **Mrs. Brown** | Oh, yes, they have always been exposed to various international foods. After leaving the hospital, I'd like to take them to our favorite sushi restaurant. |
| **Nurse** | Then, let's work together on your rehabilitation. |
| **Mrs. Brown** | Sure. |

1. a fámily of órigin     2. be séparated from     3. a wónderful expérience

4. rehabilitátion

5. Whére are you fróm?

6. What's your fávorite Japanése fóod?

7. Hów many péople are there in your fámily?

1. 相手に質問するときの表現

(Please) tell me about your family.　ご家族について話してください

Do you mind if/Would you mind if I ask you about your favorite music?
お好きな音楽について伺ってもよろしいですか.

(Yes-No Questions)

Do you have a family with you here in Japan?
ご家族は一緒に日本にお住まいですか.

Do you live alone?　お一人でお住まいですか.

(WH-Questions：what, who, when, where, how)

What is your favorite Japanese food?　お好きな日本食は何ですか.

When did you come to Japan?　いつ日本に来られたのですか.

How do you spend your holidays?　休日はどのようにお過ごしですか.

2. 相手の発言への共感を示す表現

That's wonderful. 素晴らしい.　That sounds good. いいですね.

That sounds tough. 大変そうですね.　That's too bad. 残念ですね.

(I'm) glad to hear that.　それを伺って嬉しいです.

(I'm) happy for you.　よかった.

(I'm) sorry to hear that.／Sorry for you.　お気の毒に.

3. 会話を広げたり，話題を変えたいときの表現

Speaking of curry, which do you prefer, Indian curry or Japanese curry?
カレーと言えば，インド風カレーと日本のカレーとどちらが好きですか.

When it comes to sushi, I know a good sushi restaurant nearby.
お寿司と言えば，この近くで美味しいお寿司屋さんを知っていますよ.

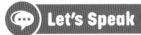 

**A.** *Interview your partner and obtain some information. Fill out the chart below. While you are asking questions, your partner should close her/his textbook. After you have finished, exchange roles with her/him.*

Your partner's name : _____

1. Hometown : She/He is from _____ .

2. Current Residence : She/He lives _____ .

3. People who she/he lives with : She/He lives _____ .
   ☐ alone   ☐ with her/his family   ☐ with her/his roommate
   ☐ _____

4. Number of people in family : There are _____ people in her/his family.
   They are _____ .   ☐ father   ☐ mother   ☐ brother(s)
   ☐ sister(s)   ☐ grandparent(s)   ☐ _____

5. Things to do in free time : She/He likes _____ .
   ☐ playing sports/online games   ☐ reading books   ☐ watching movies
   ☐ _____

6. Favorite music : Her/His favorite music is _____ .
   ☐ Japanese pop   ☐ British rock   ☐ classical music   ☐ _____

7. Favorite food : Her/His favorite food is ① _____ and her/his
   most favorite dish is ② _____ .
   ① ☐ Japanese food   ☐ Italian food   ☐ Korean food   ☐ ethnic food
      ☐ _____
   ② ☐ Japanese Ramen   ☐ pizza   ☐ Korean barbeque   ☐ Thai curry
      ☐ _____

8. Favorite place she/he's visited : Her/His favorite place is _____ ,
   because _____ .
   because ☐ she/he enjoyed the beautiful scenery   ☐ the food was terrific
   ☐ people were friendly   ☐ she/he had an interesting experience

☐ _____

Any Other Information: _____

(e.g. She/He works part-time at a restaurant./She/He keeps two cats at home./
She's/He's been so busy, having no time to relax./She/He is planning to go to
Canada next month.)

. . . . . . . . . . . . . . . . . . . . . . . . . . . . . . . . . . . . . . . . . . . . . . . . . . . . . . . . . . . . . . . . .

**B.** *Imagine that you have a patient who was admitted to the hospital
yesterday. With your partner, construct a conversation between a nurse
and a patient to get to know more about each other and practice in pairs.*

Conversation starter : Do you have a family in Japan?

Tell me about your family.

Where are you from?

What's your favorite Japanese food?

What do you do in your free time?

## Common Abbreviations

| | | |
|---|---|---|
| ADL | actívities of dáily líving | 日常生活動作 |
| AIDS | acquíred immunodefíciency sỳndrome | 後天性免疫不全症候群 |
| BM〔bm〕 | bówel mòvement | 便通，排便 |
| BP | blóod prèssure | 血圧 |
| CCU | córonary cáre ùnit | 冠疾患集中治療室〔部〕 |
| CT | compúterized tomógraphy | コンピュータ断層撮影 |
| D/C〔dc〕 | discontínue | 中止する；dischárge　退院する |
| EKG〔ECG〕 | electrocárdiogram | 心電図 |
| ER | emérgency ròom | 救急外来，救急室 |
| F | Fáhrenheit | 華氏　❶温度の単位 |
| GTT | glúcose tòlerance tèst | ブドウ糖負荷試験 |
| h, hr | hóur | 時間 |
| HR | héart ràte | 心拍数 |
| ICU | inténsive cáre ùnit | 集中治療室〔部〕，集中ケア病棟 |
| I & O | íntake and óutput | 摂取量と排泄量 |
| IV | intravénous | 静脈内の，点滴（装置） |
| lab | láboratory | 検査室 |
| MRI | magnétic résonance ìmaging | 磁気共鳴画像法 |
| OR | óperating ròom | 手術室 |
| P | púlse | 脈拍 |
| PE | phýsical examinátion | 身体診察 |
| POS | próblem-óriented sỳstem | 問題志向型システム |
| QOL | quálity of lífe | 生活の質 |
| RN | régistered núrse | 登録看護師 |
| ROM | ránge of mótion | 可動域 |
| RR | réspiratory ráte | 呼吸数 |
| T〔temp〕 | témperature | 温度，体温 |
| TB | tubèrculósis | 結核 |
| TPR | témperature, púlse, respirátion | 体温，脈拍，呼吸 |

*Spell out the following abbreviations and write the definition in Japanese.*

1. ICU
2. POS
3. ADL
4. T
5. CT
6. BP
7. AIDS
8. ROM
9. lab
10. HR
11. TB
12. QOL
13. IV
14. BM
15. OR

## 1. Length

　　1 in = 2.540 cm

　　1 cm = 0.3937 in

　　12 in = 1 ft（30.48 cm）

## 2. Weight

　　1 kg = 2.205 lb

　　1 oz = 28.35 g

　　1 lb = 16 oz（0.4536 kg）

## 3. Temperature

　　℃ =（F − 32）× 5/9

　　°F =（℃ × 1.8）+ 32

　　温度の単位には摂氏（Celsius）と華氏（Fahrenheit）があり，アメリカでは体温・気温ともに普通 Fahrenheit を用いる．98 °F は ninety-eight degrees Fahrenheit と読む．目安として次の温度を覚えておくとよい．

　　37℃ = 98.6 °F

　　0℃ = 32 °F

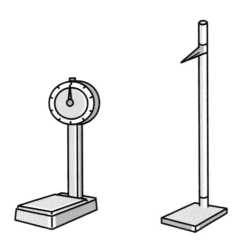

# 索引
## Glossary

84

85